I0435569

SEX
CHOCOLATE
CRY

HOW TO STAY HAPPY DURING YOUR MENSTRUAL CYCLE

BY

TAIECE LANIER AND YETUNDE TAIWO

DEDICATION

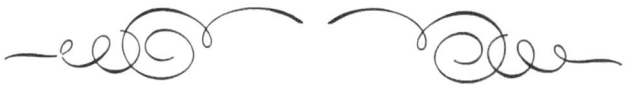

Dedicated to all the women who are suffering from their monthly visits from "AUNT FLOW", and need support getting through those irritated feelings, sweet cravings, unexpected boo-hoo moments, cramps, bloating, back pains, eating everything in sight, wishing someone would mess with you just so you could check them and the craving for sex.

We use our experiences and humor to help us get through our menstrual cycle. ENJOY!

THE INTRODUCTION

Many men have no compassion for us when it comes to "Aunt FLOW". They cannot understand how after so many years of having the same kind of pain; we are still creating a fuss about it every damn month. Yet, most of them cannot stand seeing us in pain. On average, most girls start their periods at age 12-13.

That means on average, "Aunt FLOW" Will visit you at least 456 times in your womanly lifetime. FUN! WE THINK NOT. Let's step into a humorous way of getting through those few days a month, where life just seems bloated.

Table of Contents

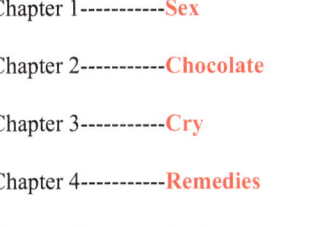

1

SEX

It's funny how horny a woman can get when she is on her period. I find that if I have more sex the week my period is to arrive, I do not experience half as much pain as I usually do.

Having sex before your period can cause you to cramp less, and if it doesn't, who cares hopefully it was great sex and all worth it.

I'm not sure why, but during my menstrual cycle my hormones rage! I want sex, sex and more sex. I find that women have mixed feelings on this topic. Some say oh no, I would never have sex on my cycle, that's just nasty, and others feel like it's even better when on their period. Having sex is way better while your "Aunt FLOW" is in town. Just add a fresh towel to your experience and enjoy!

If you're going to have sex while "Aunt FLOW" is in town, you must always carry your jet-setting period hobo handbag. This should include the following: Towel, Cotton Panties, Pony Tail Holder (if applicable), Lovin Swipes (cucumber is a favorite), Body Wash, Midol, Tea Bags, tissues and chocolate.

Some women are comfortable having sex during their period. It's not for everybody. I have heard that many men don't care, they just want to have sex, so lay a towel, get a condom and get your groove on.

It's okay to have sex while on your menstrual cycle as long as you REALLY like him. Having sex while on your cycle brings you closer to the guy. If he is just a fly by night, don't have sex while on your "PERIOD".

Your guy always knows when 'Aunt FLOW" is coming to town, because your sexy lace thongs turn into 100 percent cotton bloomer. Ouu, SEXY! NOT.

You want to have sex with him and yell at him at the same time. Oh! The conundrum.

Don't get hung up on your period. If you were an acrobat before don't stop now! Your man still wants to resume all positions.

Your breasts get plump, and that bra just looks extra sexy and all of a sudden, more guys say hi to you or look at you because you look so sexy. Meanwhile, you feel like crap and probably want to snap their heads off for even looking at you.

If you're cramping, drink something warm like tea before you start having sex, if you're not a tea girl, a shot
of vodka will do. This will normally make you feel better
and relax you. Nobody wants a cranky sex partner.

You will find that your desire for the opposite sex is
heightened. Do not be alarmed if the visions of sexing
your X pops up. It means nothing. I repeat, it means
nothing. DO NOT CALL HIM. You'll regret it the next
day.

Using your toys on your clitoris can ease the sexual energy. Get it done. Release those endorphins. You'll feel better, even if it's just for 10 minutes after, then you can go back to nursing that darn cramp, oh! The pain.

Listening to a sexy voice, even on the phone can turn you on. Feel free to indulge in the fantasy, the endorphins will do you good.

I'm so irritated, I'd rather have a toy tonight, I'm in control, no talking, no breathing, get it done and move on, don't take it personal love, I'll be fine in a few days.

Sex, sex, sex, it's all you can think of. Wondering why you are so horny? Eh! "Aunt FLOW" is heading our way, get that sex time in before she shows up, HURRY.

You're finally going to get some sex from the man you've been dating for months. You just had passionate kisses, all your hormones are raging and you head to the bathroom to take a deep breathe before your anticipated sexcapade and guess what '"Aunt FLOW" says HELLO YOU, I'm here. DAMMIT "Aunt FLOW".

You got chocolate, dessert and dozens of roses for your "beau-niversary", you're looking forward to an amazing anniversary sex and "Aunt FLOW" knocks on the door. ARE YOU KIDDING? TODAY, REALLY?

2

CHOCOLATE

My goodness sometimes chocolate is better than sex, excuse me, what am I saying, CHOCOLATE is better than sex. There is something to be said about eating chocolate during "Aunt FLOW'S" visit that just makes the world look better and feel warm and fuzzy on the inside.

I can always tell when my period is coming because I crave nothing but chocolate, wait, that's always!

How about you sit down to watch TV and you keep breaking that chocolate piece, and then you go to get another piece and realize you ran through that full Hershey's bar in less than 10 Seconds. Feel guilty much! Yah, guilt can suck it! That tasted scrumptious.

My first day is always the worst day, rolled up in my bed, fetal position, heating pad, hair in a high bun and indulging in Godiva covered chocolate strawberries to ease the pain.

If I could chow down spoons of sugar, I would but that's actually bad for you, so I eat some pink grapefruit and baptize it with sugar, then I don't feel so bad.

Wait, I just ate 2lbs of Hershey's covered almonds during commercials! But I'm on a diet, uhhhh the period life! Whyyyyyyy?

Try taking a drive when "Aunt FLOW" is heading into town, you'll find yourself buying everything you crave. They say never go to the grocery store when you are hungry. How about never go shopping when you are hungry and "Aunt FLOW" is headed to town. I once bought chickpeas from a period craving. Are you kidding me? Chickpeas? Why? Just because "Aunt FLOW" may want some. Oh! by the way it's still in the pantry months later.

The ice cream industry stays in business because of us. Are you kidding me! I eat 2 tubs of ice cream with no intention to share. Guilt? HECK NO!

I drove 10 miles for a Krispy Kreme craving and finished the 12 fresh, sizzling hot donuts in an hour. YEAH! Don't judge me

I shut down for 2 days when "Aunt FLOW" comes to town, reschedule appointments, cancel dates and turn off the phone, the only thing I want to do is eat my chocolate in peace.

I once ate a box of 24 mini cupcakes within 45 minutes, while I was driving. By the time I got home, I simply threw the box in the trash and assumed a fetal position with a cup of tea.

I ask my guy to buy me dark chocolate, and he brings back milk chocolate." What is this?" Take it back. That's one thing I don't play with, it's my chocolate!

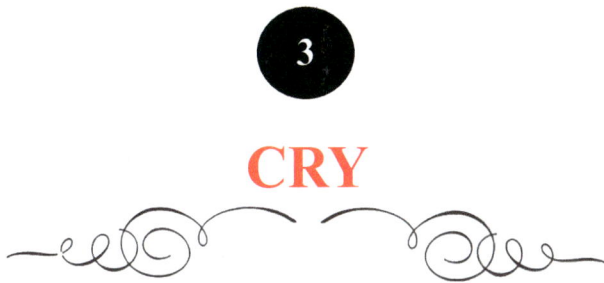

3

CRY

I just feel like crying for no damn reason.

I once cried from getting a hug. I lied and said I was just happy. It was damn "Aunt FLOW".

I'm in the store and the lady in front of me doesn't have a price on her item, the cashier calls for a price check and I just want to cry! I have my chocolate, wine and Midol in hand and all I want to do is go home! My eyes started tearing up, emotional wreck!

I was driving in my car listening to Mary Mary's 'Shackles' and broke down in tears. I mean boo-hoo ugly cry, so much so, a driver next to me asked if I was okay to which I replied through tears, "I will be okay, thank you." Thanks a lot "Aunt FLOW".

After 24 years I still don't understand how can my stomach be flat one day and look 4 months pregnant the next. I even have clothes for this time of the month, oh no, not maternity wear but "Aunt FLOW" couture. I wear maxi dresses that are comfortable and allow room for my new figure. I'm pregnant every month the only difference is the pain never stops even after 18 years.

I feel fat, ugly and un-sociable during my period. Your girlfriends should understand your desire to be a party pooper and bail frequently.

Don't go shopping on your period nothing you wear is going to look good. Trust me

Just recently I snapped at a GoDaddy phone representative because he sounded rude. I had one of those "I wish you would mess with me" moments. I felt bad, but only after "Aunt FLOW" left.

We feel so powerful and fearless and almost want to dare someone to say something to us, so we can put him or her in CHECK. Ah I love that fearless feeling. The Wrath of a woman on her period. HA!

Crying and looking at yourself in the mirror while giving an ugly cry, and seeing how you look, then crying some more. Ah! the release.

That PERIOD headache that it seems even Midol won't help with. My God, who decided this would be a sign for hormone imbalance. Dammit "Aunt FLOW".

When your guy doesn't want to see you in pain, in an effort to help, he does this.

Love you,
So here is a love-offering.
Take care until I return

—J

Normally I wouldn't care if you didn't call me, but today I do. That's "Aunt FLOW" again taking me on an emotional roller coaster.

If I don't normally text you, and you just randomly get an emotional text from me, saying "I miss you" or asking "when am I going to see you again", be suspicious. Please ignore it! Tomorrow I won't mean a word I said, that's "Aunt FLOW" talking.

Realize that if any woman is being bitchy, she may be about to receive a bag of cramps from "Aunt FLOW". Ease up on your response to her. Seriously, don't take it personally.

I find that all of a sudden cute little creatures are the most beautiful and most wonderful of God's creations, but if I catch a bug in my house when I am sitting comfy eating my chocolate, while waiting for "Aunt FLOW", Oh! It's going to die, or double die. Then, I cry for killing a living creature. Darn it "Aunt FLOW" ugh!

The irritability is off the scale, my goodness if someone said "hi" to me funny I would analyze what that "sound of hi" really meant. Are you serious? Get out of here with that fatigue "Aunt FLOW".

You feel like opening your brain and pulling out the headache spot then putting it right back.

DO NOT WORRY about the extra weight you gain at that time. Embrace it. It is a part of the cycle, the sooner you get used to it, the better for you.

Hello PPP, YES! Pre and Post Pimples, "Aunt FLOW" wants to make sure the whole world knows she is visiting you, so she gives you loads of dots to sprinkle all over your lovely face. BEAUTIFUL, just BEAUTIFUL.

Why does a pimple show up right on your forehead the night before a big date it's like saying "hey over here", "Aunt FLOW" is coming to town, want to meet her?" *Rolls eyeballs*

You will probably feel like Mother Theresa and feel EVERYTHING. Your empathy for that stray dog or raccoon in your complex becomes that of a mama goose. GET A HOLD OF YOURSELF PLEASE and remind yourself that "Aunt FLOW" is the cause of this mushiness.

A period is like having a baby, except you never have it. I'll rather have a baby every 9 months than to go through a cycle every flipping month for the next 40 plus years. DARN IT "Aunt FLOW"

My guy invites me on a trip to Antigua and I am super excited and then he gives me the dates. GAWDAMIT it's the blackout travel dates "Aunt FLOW" is scheduled to arrive. Instead of being on a beautiful island sipping on Piña coladas, I will be at home, in bed assuming a fetal position.

"Aunt FLOW" shows up sooner than expected. You're trapped outside and now asking everyone for tampons or pads. Now the whole world knows who's in town. THANKS MUCH "Aunt FLOW"

So, how do you stay happy during your menstrual cycle? Have sex, eat all the chocolate and sweet treats you want and have a good cry. You'll feel so much better. ;)

4

REMEDIES

1. Take Midol as instructed

2. Heating pads can always ease the pain for cramping

3. Force yourself to do some body stretches every morning up to 3 days before your period comes, to help for easier flow

4. Take a warm sit bath, put some Epsom salt for at least 10 minutes a day for the first 2 days.

5. Take a walk and move your body. We know you won't feel like it. DO IT ANYWAY!

6. A shot of clear liquor works

7. Get rest, since you are flowing you'll need the energy to recuperate

8. Drink more water than normal, don't worry that you will retain water, you are already bloated anyway, your body needs to stay hydrated, and it will come back to normal.

9. Take Aleve to ease the headache pressure then try to relax your mind and focus on something else, distract your mind

10. Repeat remedies 1 through 9.

5

AUTHORS

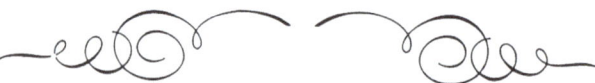

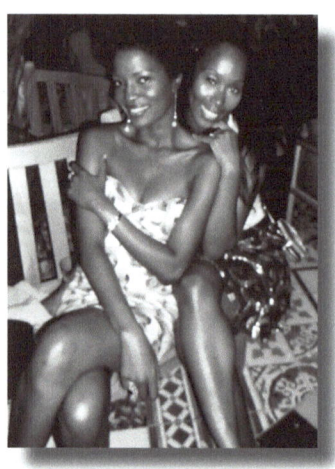

Taiece and Yetunde have been friends for over 3 years. Their passion for their Businesses/entrepreneurship and life keeps them working and living life in Sunny Miami.

This book comes from their love for living life with a side order of humor. We hope you enjoyed it.

CONNECT WITH TAIECE
www.closeteditors.com
Twitter: @closeteditors
Facebook: Closet Editors Agency
Instagram: Closeteditors

CONNECT WITH YETUNDE
www.icypr.com | www.afropolitanchef.com
Twitter: @yetunde | @afropolitanchef
Facebook: youaskicy | AfropolitanChef
Instagram: ASKICY | AfropolitanChef

6

SPECIAL BONUS OFFER FREE!!!
LOG ON TO

www.sexchocolatecry.com/special

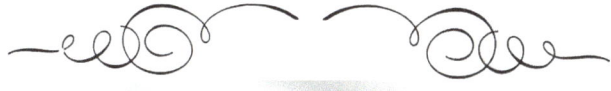

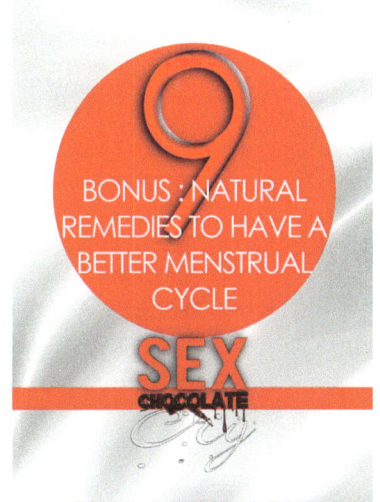

7

You and your own Sex Chocolate Cry experience.

***LET US KNOW WHAT YOU THINK ***

So how was that? Bring back any thoughts of your own experience? We hope so, and we hope it made you laugh. We would appreciate a review on our amazon page. Do feel free to share your thoughts on Facebook and Twitter with your friends and fans. If you believe the book is worth sharing with your girlfriends, please would you take a few seconds to let them know about it? If it turns out to make a difference in their sexy, chocolate filled lives, they'll be forever grateful to you, as will we.

For now, go have some safe sex, eat that chocolate and have a good merry cry. "Aunt FLOW" can't do anything about it.

CONNECT ONLINE: FIND US AT

WWW.SEXCHOCOLATECRY.COM

FACEBOOK:

WWW.FACEBOOK.COM/SEXCHOCOLATECRY

TWITTER:

WWW.TWITTER.COM/SEXCHOCOLATECRY

INSTAGRAM:

WWW.INSTAGRAM.COM/SEXCHOCOLATECRY

SEX
CHOCOLATE
CRY
HOW TO STAY HAPPY DURING YOUR MENSTRUAL CYCLE

BY

TAIECE LANIER AND YETUNDE TAIWO

THANK YOU